Healing Shingle　　　　　　　　　　—puthic Pain

By
Lynne D M Noble

Copyright 2018 Lynne D M Noble

This book shall not, by way of trade or otherwise, be lent, re-sold, hired out, or otherwise circulated without the prior consent of the copyright holder or the publisher in any form of binding or cover than that in which it is published and without a similar condition including this condition being imposed on the subsequent purchaser.
The use of its contents in another media is also subject to the same conditions.

Independently published

Independently published 2019

About the Author

Lynne Noble was born in 1953 in Huddersfield, West Yorkshire. From a very early age, Lynne showed an interest in nutrition and genetics avidly reading any books that she could get her hands on at the time.

Initially, Lynne studied orthopaedics but events led her to work with the elderly mentally infirm. Here, her interest in neurodegenerative disorders and pain syndromes developed.

Lynne undertook rigorous programmes of study, completing her Cert Ed., (FE) BSc (Hons) and Adv. Dip Education simultaneously before moving onto her M.Ed.

From there she took further demanding programmes in Human Nutrition, Pharmacology, Neuroscience, Genetics and Immunology. During this time, she was given many prestigious awards for her academic work. It was noted then that Lynne was not afraid of tackling difficult subjects.

She began her law degree but ill health prevented her from pursuing this. However, in this time, she moved from being a foster parent to adoptive parent.

She has been instrumental in setting up projects in the community for disadvantaged groups.

She is a member of the Guild of Health Writers and a member of the British Union of Journalists.

Now retired, she lives in a picturesque village in West Yorkshire with her husband. She enjoys gardening, watching her husband bowling and researching.

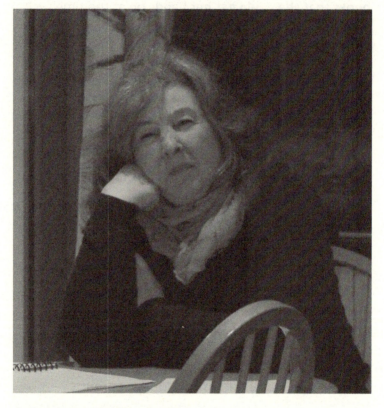

Author Lynne Noble at home

https://quintessentiallylynne.weebly.com/nutritional-medicine.html

Contents

Preface

My grandfather fought in the Great War. He lost his younger brother in that war. He also lost all his friends in that war when they froze to death, huddled together. My grandfather was the only one to survive. He battled diphtheria and won. He married the love of his life but had to give up his business when my grandmother became ill and was unable to help him. He lost his youngest son, my father, when my father was only thirty-seven. My grandfather lived through many hardships and he dealt with them all with strength, love and humour .... well, apart from one and that is when he got a bout of shingles at the age of eighty-nine.

Within weeks, he had contracted pneumonia, no doubt helped along by the fact that the pain, from shingles, was so bad, that he was unable to eat.

It was a quick decline. I lost my much loved grandfather to a childhood virus that lays dormant, until it is safe for it to rear its ugly head and wreak havoc on unsuspecting people.

That was really my first introduction to nerve pain and how debilitating it is – more so because conventional painkillers, such as ibuprofen and paracetamol do not work on neuropathic pain.

Neuropathic pain is relentless. It destroys sleep, quality of life, relationships and ………. there is no knowing if, or when, it will end.

Given the impact that shingles has on people's lives, I am surprised that few people know how debilitating it can be. Whenever I meet someone they tell me that they have shingles or have recently had it. They are still in pain. They are beside themselves with pain but nothing will shift it.

There are some medications which deal with neuropathic pain but they are not always prescribed and they do carry marked side effects. The side effects can reduce your quality of life in other ways so you may have to decide, on balance, whether the pain is worse than the side effects of taking medication.

Some people, who have been inoculated against shingles, still get it; sometimes more than once. However, it is still recommended that you are inoculated against it as the first line of defence. If the virus lying dormant in your system, still awakens to wreak its havoc on your nerves, then a timely trip to the GP is required for an antiviral medication which should shorten the life of the attack.

It is hoped that this will mean less damage to the nerves which have been attacked by the virus.

Prevention is a far better aim. The shingles virus does not rear its ugly head until the immune system is below par but if it is already too late to prevent shingles then we need to know what we can do about the symptoms as well as cut short the attack.

If the pain is still evident then we need to look at nutrients which can firstly, help heal the damage to the nerves and secondly, repair the damaged nerve.

Nerves take a long time to heal, so pain relief is a must while they are doing so.

I think that I should add that attention must be made to diet, too. Shingles is an opportunistic infection and waits until the immune system is weakened before mounting its attack.

I have seen far too many people suffer because of the effects of this illness. Hence why this book had to be written.

Close to home

My brother-in-law always rang on a Sunday evening to speak to my husband. One Sunday, when he rang, he sounded very ill indeed. This was unusual for he was never ill. He was as fit as a fiddle even though he was in his seventies.

He reported that during the week he had felt unusually shivery, hot and extremely unwell. He felt so ill that he sat in his armchair for a couple of days, not eating or drinking or caring for himself at all.

He would have been there even longer if a friend had not popped by and urged him to go to the doctor. My brother-in-law had not thought of this for some reason. Nevertheless, he took himself off to see a GP and was diagnosed with shingles. The rash had snaked itself across his face and eye. He could have lost his sight if his friend had not popped by and urged him to see a doctor.

My brother-in-law was given antiviral medication and lived to tell the tale but the memory of the intensity of the pain and just how ill he was, at the time, have not left him.

I don't know of anybody for whom this is not true but what is shingles and why does it cause so much pain? It is to this that we will now turn.

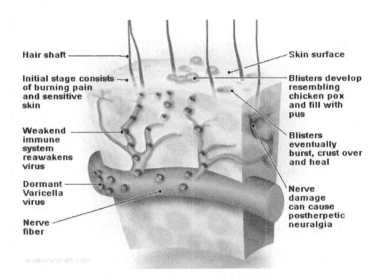

Hair shaft

Initial stage consists of burning pain and sensitive skin

Weakend immune system reawakens virus

Dormant Varicella virus

Nerve fiber

Skin surface

Blisters develop resembling chicken pox and fill with pus

Blisters eventually burst, crust over and heal

Nerve damage can cause postherpetic neuralgia

¹Diagram showing the impact of the Varicella virus

¹ https://www.graceer.com/shingles/

What is Shingles?

Shingles is a viral infection that is caused by the varicella-zoster virus. This is the same virus that causes chicken pox. After you have had chicken pox, the virus lies dormant in nerve tissue. This is a survival strategy by the virus. Immune system cells could wipe out the virus but it would destroy nervous tissue and this could have devastating effects. The most the immune system will do is keep the virus in check until the immune system is compromised and the virus is reactivated.

Once the virus is reactivated, it generally appears as a stripe of blisters which follows the line of the nerve it has been hiding in. Normally, it affects one side of your torso but it can affect the face and area around your eyes. The latter is an emergency. Shingles can cause blindness if it attacks nerves supplying the eye.

Early symptoms of shingles

- Burning pain and sensitive skin
- The appearance of blisters
- The blisters crusting over after bursting
- Post herpetic neuralgia

People may also have:

- Fever
- Sensitivity to light
- Headache
- Extreme fatigue

What is post herpetic neuralgia?

Post herpetic pain is chronic pain which runs along the cutaneous nerves. The pain is often distorted.

The pain can be described in a number of ways:

- Sharp and jabbing
- Burning
- Deep and achy

People with neuralgia often have allodynia. Allodynia is a condition which causes extreme sensitivity to pain. People with this condition cannot bear even the slightest touch of clothing on their skin.

When nerve damage occurs the outer coating of the nerve, the myelin sheath, is attacked. This means that nerve impulses, which carry messages, are not able to carry out their function. This leads to the intense pain which is felt in shingles.

Diagram showing transmission of messages carried from one nerve to the next

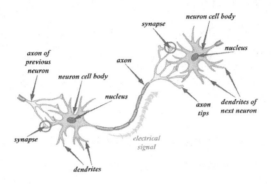

2

How do we help to repair the damaged nerve and heal the pain?

Nerves take a notoriously long time to heal but they cannot do it at all without some vital nutrients, some of which also help to attenuate the pain.

2 http://simplebiologyy.blogspot.com/2014/08/conduction-of-nerve-impulse.html

As we have discussed, in normal circumstances cell mediated immunity continually suppresses the virus responsible for shingles. As aging progresses, there are a number of nutritional deficiencies as well as many other medical conditions which are a risk factor for reactivation of the virus. These risk factors include:

- Chronic obstructive pulmonary disease
- Inflammatory bowel disease
- Immunosuppressive therapy
- Chemotherapy
- Rheumatic diseases

Micronutrient deficiency is a risk factor for cell mediated immunity dysfunction and therefore also a risk factor for the reactivation of the shingles virus.

We will now look at some of these substances and how they help the healing of neuropathic pain.

Alpha Lipoic Acid

Alpha lipoic acid (ALA) is a special type of antioxidant. Antioxidants help prevent damage to the body's cells.

ALA is made naturally in the body, although its synthesis lessens as we age. It is a special antioxidant in that it is both fat and water soluble. This means it can have a positive effect anywhere in the body. It also helps the body to produce other antioxidants, when required.

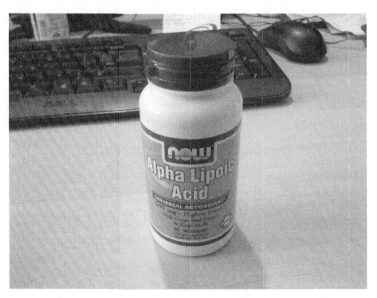

ALA is able to pass into the brain, quite easily. This means that it can help to ameliorate any damage to brain cells.

A number of studies, conducted in Germany, have demonstrated the beneficial effects of ALA on nerves.

1258 participants were given 600mg of ALA, intravenously. It was reported that the patients who received ALA in this way, had a marked improvement in their nerve pain, within three weeks.

It was found that a daily dose of 600mg worked just as well as higher doses.

Of course, you do not have to wait until you get shingles to start increasing the amount of ALA in your diet. It is a marvellous nutrient and attention should be paid in incorporating it into your diet on a regular basis.

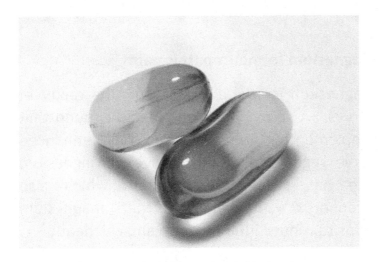

Alpha lipoic acid is a fat and water soluble nutrient

Where is ALA found?

The highest amounts of ALA can be found in

- Brewers' yeast
- Liver
- Red meat

Good vegetarian sources are:

- Broccoli
- spinach

Magnesium for neuropathic pain

Magnesium is a vital nutrient for the repair of nerves. A study[3] published in 2011 found that supplementing with magnesium enhanced nerve regeneration and recovery. Magnesium also has an inhibitory action which also attenuates pain signals. Further, magnesium helps to reduce inflammation and cell death.

How does magnesium inhibit pain?

N-methyl -D-aspartate (NMDA) is a receptor for the neurotransmitter, glutamate. This means that a tiny part on brain cells is able to attach itself to a chemical called glutamate. Once glutamate has attached itself to the receptor it activates it. Glycine and serine, which are amino acids, may also activate the NMDA receptors.

However, glycine does have a pain inhibitory and anti-anxiety action through different channels. As it can activate or inhibit it may be useful in some individuals and not others.

---

[3] https://www.ncbi.nlm.nih.gov/pubmed/21609904

When the NMDA receptors are activated they are associated with increased non-neuropathic pain, neuropathic pain. They also reduce the function of opioid receptors. This means that the receptors that are attracted to the pain killing opioids do not work as well. However, the level of activity on this this type of receptor varies.

What you need to remember is that when the NMDA receptors are activated then there is increased pain and opioid drugs do not work as well.

Common prescription opioids are:

- morphine
- codeine

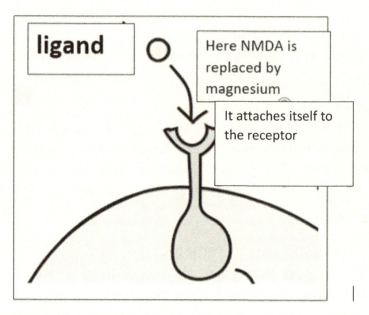

Magnesium is an antagonist of NMDA and can stop the receptor from being activated

Over activation of the NMDA receptor is relieved by magnesium as it causes a block on excessive influx of calcium ions that lead to excitotoxicity and increased pain levels.

However, it is important to preserve some NMDA receptor activity; we only want to remove **excessive** activity. In effect what is required is that the NMDA receptor is activated and then a channel blocker (also known as an uncompetitive receptor antagonist) blocks the flow of calcium ions that increase pain levels.

In medicine, the drugs ketamine, amantadine and memantine are prescribed as NMDA blockers.

However, they have some horrible side effects. For example, Amantadine can cause projectile vomiting within minutes of it being taken.

Insomnia, drowsiness, headache, constipation and blurred vision are but of the other reported side effects.

. However, there are a number of natural NMDA receptor blockers which do not have these negative reactions and these include:

- parsley (contains agipenin)
- zinc (NMDA antagonist)
- garlic (s-aldyl cysteine)
- Dimethyl sulfoxide (DMSO) (an NMDA antagonist)

These substances are all found in local supermarkets or can be obtained in health food stores or online.

Recipes for pain relieving shots can be found at the end of this book.

Nerve repair

A study[4] published in 2011 found that supplementing with magnesium improved neurological recovery and enhanced nerve regeneration.

Magnesium has long been known to help nerves repair themselves, reduce inflammation and inhibit cell death. Consequently, this helps nerve function to be restored.

Magnesium is found in dark green, leafy vegetables, legumes, sea food and nuts.

If supplementing with magnesium then 500mg daily is recommended especially if the patient is taking diuretics or laxatives, when magnesium is easily lost in excessive urination.

Magnesium tablets are easy to source and are generally available on supermarket shelves at a very reasonable price.

_____

[4] https://www.ncbi.nlm.nih.gov/pmc/articles/PMC5270442/

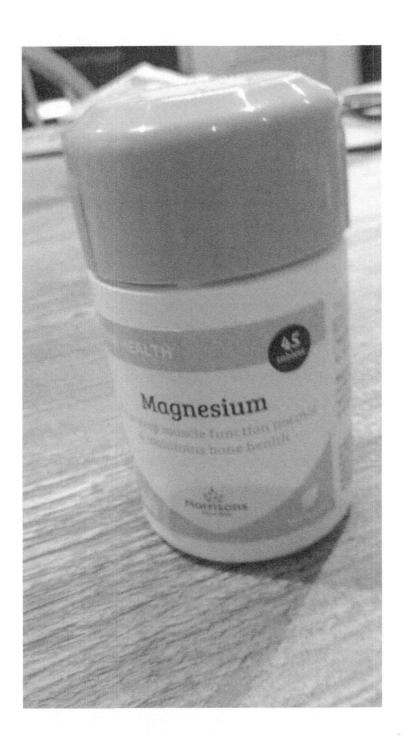

Magnesium can also be added to bath water in the form of magnesium sulphate (Epsom Salts). Magnesium oil can be applied directly to any areas of neuropathic pain and left for at least 30 minutes before being wiped off. It is able to penetrate the skin quite easily.

Alternatively, if the area of pain can be wrapped in cling film after the magnesium oil has been applied then this allows it to sink even further.

DMSO is a carrier and will help the deeper penetration of magnesium oil. Apply the magnesium oil to clean skin and then massage in the DMSO. Wash off with warm water twenty minutes later. (DMSO will be looked at in more detail later).

Vitamin D

A deficiency of vitamin D is known to cause widespread pain. The greater the vitamin D deficiency the worse nerve damage there is. Further, a deficiency of vitamin D lowers the pain threshold.

A study[5] of the relationship between vitamin D and neuropathy found that vitamin D levels were inversely proportional to neuropathy symptoms score.

Most people are deficient in vitamin D. As it is difficult to obtain from food then I recommend a supplement even though vitamin D can be synthesised from the action of the sun's rays on the skin.

Absorption of nutrients and synthesis of vitamin D, from cholesterol, is less efficient as we age.

Whenever someone has shingles I would always recommend a test for vitamin D deficiency.

---

[5] https://www.ncbi.nlm.nih.gov/pubmed/22284260

Vitamin D is so bound up in the smooth working of the immune system that shingles is an indicator that there is insufficient vitamin D in the system.

It is practically impossible to get enough vitamin D from the diet. There are few sources. These include:

- Oily fish – mackerel and sardines, for example
- Irradiated mushrooms – that is mushrooms that have been left out in the sun
- Beef liver
- Fortified products like some dairy products and cereals
- Egg yolks

Foods containing vitamin D need to be taken with a little fat in order for it to be absorbed.

An egg yolk contains about 220 International Units of vitamin D.

The recommended dietary allowance for vitamin D which was set in the 1950's is 400 IU's. This is far too low since this was set at this level in order to avoid rickets only. It is not enough to maintain health. More and more researchers are now revising this figure upwards to 2000 IU's daily.

Sunlight does help the synthesis of vitamin D but there isn't enough sunlight in the winter months for this to occur.

In addition, cholesterol is needed to synthesise vitamin D so statin users may be at particular risk of viral infections like shingles.

Even if supplementation is not necessary in the summer, it is very likely that it is needed in the winter. In addition, those groups of people with intestinal absorption problems, dark skin, poor diets or who live indoors most of the time are still likely to need supplementation of vitamin D in the summer months.

Vitamin C and other micronutrients

Studies[6] have shown a weak dose response relationship between decreasing levels of vitamin C and increasing levels of herpes zoster in all participants. A similar relationship is found in those with a lower iron intake.

A strong dose response association was found between the decreased risk of activating herpes zoster with a higher intake of seven micronutrients which included vitamins A, B, C, E, folic acid, zinc and iron. Such a mix was found to possess significant antiviral effects.

Other studies[7] have found that high intravenous vitamin C rapidly reduces the blistering and skin rashes found in shingles. It has also been found to reduce acute herpetic pain.

---

[6] Thomas SL, Wheeler JG, Hall AJ. Micronutrient intake and the risk of herpes zoster: a case-control study. Int J Epidemiol. 2006;35:307–314

[7] Schencking M, Sandholzer H, Frese T. Intravenous administration of vitamin C in the treatment of herpetic neuralgia:two case reports. Med Sci Monit. 2010;16:CS58–61.

In the apparently healthy elderly, deficiencies of zinc and vitamin C are ranked as the first and second major cause of micronutrient deficiencies and these deficiencies are also considered to be risk factors for herpes zoster and post herpetic neuralgia.

Zinc can be depleted by excessive intake of copper, so if you have a diet which is excessively high in copper then you may need to make some changes. However, the intention is not to attempt to completely eliminate copper from the diet. It is required to help absorb iron from the intestines.

Iron has we have already seen is one of those nutrients that helps to reduce the risk factor for shingles.

Copper serves many vital purposes in the body. It helps retain pigmentation of the hair and skin, it is part of the composition of the myelin sheath. Copper also aids the immune system.

Copper kills bacteria, viruses and fungi on contact.

However, a zinc deficiency seems to be implicated in the reactivation of the shingles virus. We are talking about a balance here.

The following foods are excellent sources of copper:[8]

	Amount	RDI
Beef liver, cooked	1 oz (28 g)	458%
Oysters, cooked	6	133%
Lobster, cooked	1 cup (145 g)	141%
Lamb liver, cooked	1 oz (28 g)	99%
Squid, cooked	3 oz (85 g)	90%
Dark chocolate	3.5 oz bar (100 g)	88%
Oats, raw	1 cup (156 g)	49%
Sesame seeds, roasted	1 oz (28 g)	35%
Cashew nuts, raw	1 oz (28 g)	31%

---

[8] https://www.healthline.com/nutrition/copper-deficiency-symptoms#section11

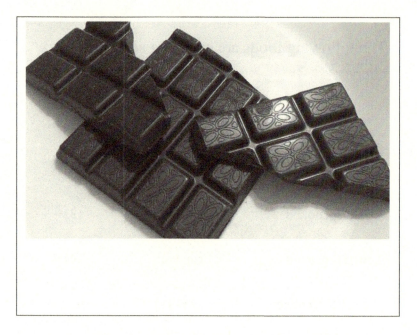

Dark chocolate contains useful amounts of copper

You can see that beef liver is very high in copper. However, beef liver is also a very good source of zinc too as well as vitamin D and A and the B vitamins. It is an excellent food for the older population.

Foods which contain high amounts of zinc are:

- Legumes
- Meat
- Dairy

- Nuts
- Seeds
- Whole grains

It might be worth looking at zinc and the role it has to play in preventing shingles and post herpetic neuralgia in a little more detail.

Zinc – a great antiviral

A study[9] of Taiwanese patients with post herpetic neuralgia found that they were deficient in the mineral, zinc.

Zinc is a trace element. This means it is only required in very small amounts in our body. In spite of this, it has a number of important roles in the body.

Zinc is required to activate T lymphocytes (T cells). T cells are important because they

- help regulate immune responses
- attack infected or cancerous cells

A study[10] found that the immune system was severely compromised due to a lack of available zinc and, in addition, zinc deficient people were susceptible to a wide range of pathogens.

---

[9]
https://www.researchgate.net/publication/51033105_Nutrient_deficiencies_as_a_risk_factor_in_Taiwanese_patients_with_postherpetic_neuralgia
[10] https://www.ncbi.nlm.nih.gov/pubmed/9701160?dopt=Abstract

The normal recommended dietary allowance of zinc is:

- 11mg for men
- 8mg for women

However, zinc can be taken in high doses (50mg) daily during a shingles outbreak. Zinc is able to inhibit the herpes zoster virus from replicating.

Good sources of zinc include:

- Meat
- Shellfish
- Beans, chickpeas, lentils and other legumes
- Eggs
- Whole grains
- Nuts
- Dairy
- Seeds

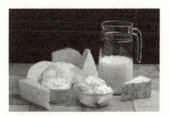

Dairy foods are good sources of zinc.

Lysine – amino acid that inhibits viral replication

Lysine inhibits the growth of the Herpes Zoster virus that causes shingles. Lysine is an essential amino acid which means that it must be obtained from food as the body does not make it.

As a preventative, lysine can be taken at a dose of 1,000mg daily

At the first sign of shingles, even before the rash erupts, take lysine at a dose of 1,000- 1,500 mg three times daily.

Good sources of dietary lysine are:

- Meat
- Cheese
- Cod and sardines
- Soybean
- spirulina

Glycine – good all round amino acid

Amino acids are the building blocks of protein and, as such are found in all animal foods. Peas, beans and other legumes are rich sources of animal protein.

Amino acids can be non–essential, that is they can be made in the body, or essential which means they must be taken in through diet. Some amino acids are also said to be conditional which means that normally the body can make them but, at times of illness or injury, they may need to be supplemented.

It would be remiss of me if I did not add glycine as one of the mainstays of the shingle sufferer's emergency kit. Not only can It can relieve intractable pain in less than a day but it can continue to employ its anti-inflammatory and analgesic properties if it is taken on a daily basis, in sufficient amounts.

Glycine is the smallest amino acid of the twenty amino acids. Only nine amino acids are classed as essential. Glycine, however, is a non-essential amino acid. This means it is capable of being synthesised from another amino acid, by the body, when needed.

The story should end there but, of course, it doesn't. Our current diets do not support the synthesis of enough glycine to support health, including our immune systems.

If we are deficient in the amino acids that go onto make glycine or we lack nutrients which help bring about this process, then we simply cannot make this, the smallest of the amino acids.

Let's look at some more of the actions of this marvellous nutritional all round amino acid.

Glycine reduces pain

Glycine is an inhibitory amino acid which means that it can inhibit pain signals. This calming influence reduces the sensation of pain.

Glycine reduces inflammation

Glycine acts directly on cells which are involved in the inflammatory process. It suppresses free radicals which are highly reactive molecules that go around – like an out of control pinball – damaging cells which get in its way. Glycine also suppresses inflammatory cytokines.

Inflammatory cytokines are molecules which are secreted from immune cells like macrophages. (Big eaters). These molecules help promote inflammation. Of course, it is the inflammatory processes which cause the pain.

Glycine blocks processes which raise inflammation

Fructose is a type of sugar commonly found in fruit. It has the ability to raise inflammation through a cell signalling molecule called Tumour Necrosis Factor (TNF). Glycine has the ability to block this process and further block another molecule called interleukin 6 which is also involved in the inflammatory process.

Where can glycine be found? Glycine is normally found in many of the foods that we don't eat nowadays. These include:

- Bone broths
- Chicken skin
- Pork scratchings
- Pigs ears
- Tripe
- Organ meats

to name but a few.

However, although glycine can inhibit pain, it can also activate the NMDA receptor in **some** people. These variations are due to genetic differences. If glycine doesn't work, leave it out but, in most cases, it does alleviate neuropathic pain.

The role of microglia in pain

The activation of microglia which are cells in the central nervous system are responsible for chronic pain [11] Microglia are the macrophages (scavengers) of the central nervous system. Studies have shown that spinal microglia were activated in response to injury of peripheral nerves.

---

[11] theconversation.com/what-causes-chronic-pain-microglia-might-be-to-blame-6173

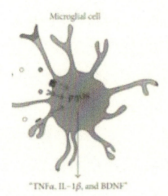
Microglial cell

"TNFα, IL-1β, and BDNF"

Spinal microglia are activated when damage to peripheral nerves happens. However, **glycine,** which we have already mentioned, inhibits the activation of microglia, thus reducing the potential for pain.

When minocycline (an antibiotic which can cross the blood brain barrier) was administered to rats it was found to prevent pain. Minocycline inhibits microglia and other cells such as astrocytes from 'cross talking' with neurons. It has been firmly established that this cross talk is necessary for the development of chronic pain.

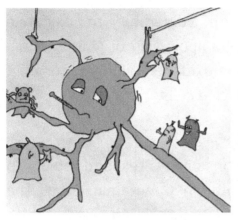

12 Microglia cross talk with brain cells this is how they develop and maintain chronic pain.

GABA (gamma amino butyric acid)

GABA acts as a brake on pain impulses. It is found in spinal nerve cells. When these GABA producing cells are damaged or die, the pain system can get out of control.

During nerve damage there is an assault by reactive oxygen services which are produced at the time of injury.

---

12 http://blog.donders.ru.nl/?p=4862&lang=en

GABA neurons are vulnerable to oxidative stress. Taking alpha lipoic acid or glutathione – both powerful antioxidants will help protect these GABA producing cells.

Vitamin C

Acute viral infections always respond rapidly to mega doses of vitamin C. Vitamin C has the ability to access all tissues in the body which enhances its effectiveness.

Pain relief, with vitamin C, has been found to take place at doses of 3000mg.

To treat the ongoing pain of shingles, take vitamin C to bowel tolerance.[13] The pain should disappear quite quickly.

Any excess vitamin C will be passed out in the urine.

Repeat if, and when, the pain returns.

---

[13] Bowel tolerance occurs when the stools become loose due to the amount of vitamin C taken. This will differ among individuals.

This mega dosing, with vitamin C, should continue until the infection and lesions have disappeared.

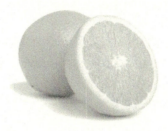

Oranges are a good source of vitamin C

Listerine (mouthwash)

Listerine, which is marketed as a mouthwash, has been used to good effect in alleviating the pain of shingles – often overnight. While the reason for this is not currently known, you do not need to know how it works, for it to work.

It is worth trying. You will not have lost anything since you can still use it as a mouthwash if application to the area, affected by shingles, is not effective.

Many of the mouthwashes on the market which help prevent gum disease will have a similar action. As such it is a useful treatment while you wait for an appointment with the GP or the receipt of prescription medication.

In addition to providing some relief they also help dry up the area affected by the virus.

However, it is probably better not used is the skin is broken.

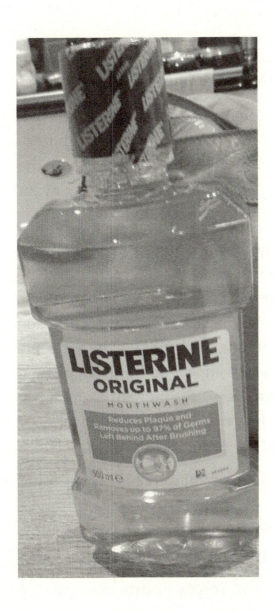

Vitamin B$_{12}$ – repairer of myelin sheath

Vitamin B$_{12}$ (Cobalamin) is a vitamin that is essential for the development and function of brain and nerve cells. It helps promote the synthesis of lecithin which is a major component of the myelin sheath lipids.

There are only animal sources of Vitamin B$_{12}$ and even then, this vitamin can only be separated from its food source in an acidic environment. Stomach acidity tends to lessen in older age. In addition, many elderly people take antacids which impact on how well vitamin B$_{12}$ can be absorbed. Further problems arise when there is loss of appetite often associated with illness and old age.

This vitamin is generally taken with other vitamins of the B complex. It is easy to source and can be found on the shelves of most supermarkets at a reasonable price.

Be guided by the dosage instructions on the container.

Lactoferrin

This is a substance produced by the body as part of the immune system defences. It is found in high amounts in colostrum and it is a powerful antiviral. Supplementing with lactoferrin strengthens the immune system.

Lactoferrin supplements are made using bovine colostrum and can be bought online or in health food stores.

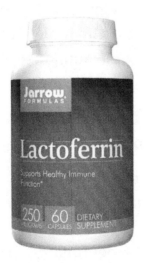

Lactoferrin is a powerful antiviral

The role of Theanine in alleviating pain

Theanine is an amino acid that is not generally found in the human diet. It is not an essential amino acid nor is it considered to be a non-essential amino acid, either.

Theanine is generally referred to as a non-dietary amino acid. It has relaxing but not sedating properties. It helps deals with stressful situations and helps improve attention. Theanine has also been found to enhance immune function.

In spite of its varied benefits it is only found in tea – either green or black.

Theanine is a blocker of substance P. Substance P is found in the spinal cord and brain and is a major player in promoting pain and inflammation including neuropathic pain. It is found in brain circuits that promote anxiety. It is not surprising that people reach for a cup of tea containing theanine, when needing to wind down.

Since the sources of theanine are limited, you have to be creative in thinking up ways to include it in the diet. Dried fruit is traditionally steeped in strong tea before being incorporated in a cake mix. However, teas slightly bitter flavour may not allow it to be incorporated into many dishes if you do not like bitter flavours in the first place.

 L-theanine can be bought relatively cheaply – considering its benefits - in most health food shops and online.

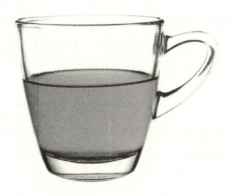

Capsaicin cream for pain

Capsaicin is a useful treatment for post herpetic neuralgia. It is a natural compound found in capsicum that is able to alleviate pain by activating and desensitising nerve fibres.

Capsaicin alleviates pain by decreasing the intensity of pain signals generated by Substance P. It is a useful adjunctive medicine to be used alongside one of the NMDA receptors.

Ready-made capsaicin creams are readily available in health food stores and online. However, these tend to be expensive.

A little dried capsaicin, incorporated into hog fat and rubbed into the affected area will do just as good a job as proprietary brands of capsaicin cream for far less cost.

If you like the spiciness of capsaicin and can incorporate it into your diet on a fairly regular basis this will also help reduce neuropathic pain.

Capsaicin should be applied to the skin three to four times daily. Initially, the application may cause a burning sensation but this will dissipate quite quickly after application.

The treatment should be continued for at least one month.

Caution: cream should only be applied once the shingles blisters have dried and dropped off.

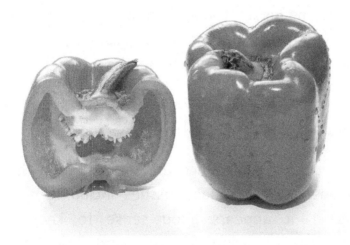

Capsaicin is useful for neuropathic pain

Nerve repair

A study published in 2011 found that supplementing with magnesium improved neurological recovery and enhanced nerve regeneration. Magnesium helps nerves repair themselves after injury. In addition, magnesium helps reduce inflammation and prevent cell death which can help restore nerve function. That means that magnesium oil doesn't just mask the symptoms of neuropathy, it can actually help your body to heal!

The medicine chest

Given the prevalence of viruses and their propensity to damage tissues including nerve tissue, it appears good sense to keep an antiviral medicine kit to hand but, more importantly, become acquainted with the properties of the components of this kit.

Viruses can wreak havoc in a short space of time and by the time the pain. or rash, has motivated the shingles sufferer to seek help from the doctor, the nerve, or nerves, will most likely have suffered a great deal of damage.

Nerves re-myelinate slowly, compared to damaged skin or intestinal cells, so it pays to respond to a shingles infection as soon as you are aware of it. The nerve coating – the myelin sheath – requires cholesterol and copper as part of its composition.

Those taking statins are 25% more likely to reactivate the shingles virus a Canadian study found.

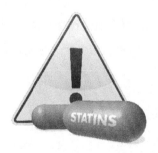

There are many studies showing that statin users have an increased risk of dying from a respiratory or gastrointestinal infection.

Statins suppress the innate immune system. In addition, cholesterol is required to help form part of the membranes of cells of the innate immune system. The innate immune system is the body's defence system that you were born with. It is clear that if cholesterol is artificially lowered it will impact on your ability to withstand infection, including shingles.

A 2018 study from South Korea[14] compared 25,726 statin users and an equal number of non-statin users. Their results mirrored the Canadian study in that there was a 25% increase in shingles virus reactivation for those taking statins. However, if the statin users were more than 70% years old then this increased risk of developing shingles rose to 39%.

----

[14]

https://journals.plos.org/plosone/article?id=10.1371/journal.pone.0198263

It is clear that shingles is better to be avoided at all costs through the administration of a single shingles vaccine. It has a high success rate but there are always some people who do not appear to respond or for whom the vaccine is only partially successful.

For those taking statins, they may wish to discuss whether they are absolutely necessary in light of increasing concerns that are emerging about statin use.

Careful attention to diet must not take a back seat. Your ability to withstand infection is closely associated with the calibre of your nutrition.

If all the above fails, then you need to be able to treat the post herpetic pain that will follow an attack of shingles. A little forethought is priceless. Rather than wait until neuropathic pain strikes, the remedies should already be to hand. Shingles strikes without warning. It may be, of course, that you are one of the lucky ones and never have an attack of shingles. The medicine chest won't be wasted, if you don't.

he nutritional substances mentioned work equally as well on non-neuropathic pain including arthritis and other inflammatory disorders.

.

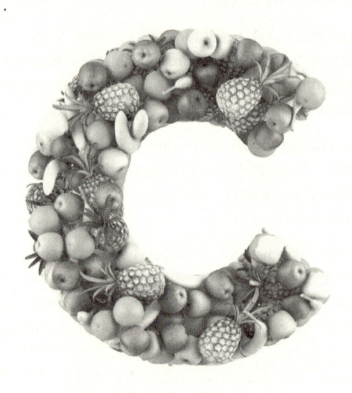

Vitamin C can shorten an attack of shingles

Pain relieving shots

Green zinger

Juice some parsley, celery and green pepper with a couple of cloves of garlic.

Drink along with supplements of:

- 400mg of magnesium and
- 15mg of zinc

Chamomile tea (contains NMDA antagonist)

Add some fresh orange if desired

Drink with 400mg of magnesium

15mg of zinc

Black or green tea also contains NMDA antagonists. Drink it strong and often.

Olive oil – use liberally on salads. Add fresh chopped herbs. lemon and garlic to the oil

Foods that contain luteolin, an NMDA receptor antagonist

Flavonoids - Flavones - Luteolin		
Oils		
Oils - Fruit vegetable oils	Olive, oil, extra virgin	0.36 mg/100 g FW
	Olive, oil, refined	0.12 mg/100 g FW
	Olive, oil, virgin	0.13 mg/100 g FW
Seasonings		
Herbs	Common sage, fresh	33.40 mg/100 g FW
	Common thyme, fresh	39.50 mg/100 g FW
	Lemon verbena, dried	4.52 mg/100 g FW
	Mexican oregano, dried	56.33 mg/100 g FW
	Rosemary, dried	3.00 mg/100 g FW
Seeds		
Nuts	Pistachio, dehulled	0.10 mg/100 g FW
Pulses - Lentils	Lentils, whole, raw	0.03 mg/100 g FW
Vegetables		
Fruit vegetables	Olive [Black], raw	3.43 mg/100 g FW
	Olive [Green], raw	0.56 mg/100 g FW
Shoot vegetables	Globe artichoke, heads, raw	42.10 mg/100 g FW

DMSO (Dimethyl Sulfoxide)

DMSO is a solvent with powerful anti-inflammatory properties. As a solvent it easily penetrates skin taking with it any other substances that are on the skin such as capsaicin cream. This would enhance the pain relieving effects of any creams and ointments that are designed for this purpose. However, it has the potential to take unwanted substances with it and application to any injured area should only be undertaken on clean skin.

However, DMSO has other qualities other than its powerful pain relieving properties. It has been found that infectious diseases respond to DMSO. During an ordinary attack of shingles, although the pain is memorable for a few days, it generally does not result in post herpetic neuralgia. When this disabling condition does occur then DMSO can respond admirably to it. Using one teaspoon of DMSO combined with one teaspoon of distilled water, this can be used to gargle with if the blisters appear in the mouth or applied over the blisters if on the skin.

DMSO solidifies if the room temperature is cold and it will need to be allowed to warm before it changes to a liquid state. It has an oily feel. Some people take small - and diluted - amounts by mouth and this is not harmful in itself although the taste is prohibitive.

DMSO is better used on the skin and washed off after it has been given skin contact for twenty minutes but may be left longer if there is unlikely to be contamination from whatever you come into contact with.

DMSO can be used with magnesium oil or capsaicin cream to enhance their pain relieving properties.

DMSO can be obtained from Amazon and some health food shops and should be labelled as 99% pure if used for medicinal purposes.

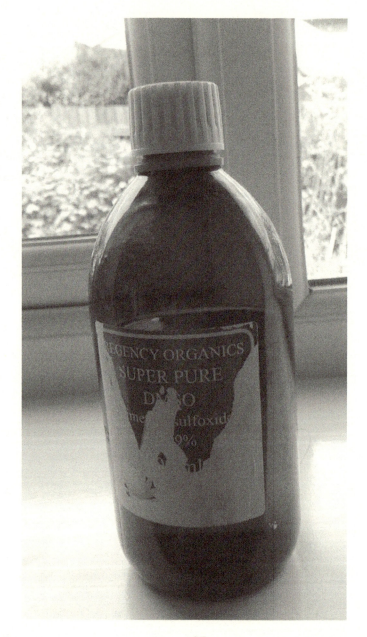

57

Adenosine

Not many people have heard of adenosine never mind know what it does. Adenosine is a regulatory molecule in metabolic processes. Therefore, it is vital for health.

In the brain, adenosine is a neurotransmitter (brain chemical) that has an inhibitory action. It promotes sleep. Levels of adenosine rise throughout the day in response to exercise. At the end of the day provided adenosine levels are high enough then arousal is suppressed and sleep promoted.

Adenosine has many other actions including energy metabolism and expenditure.

 The more physical exercise that you do the more the more adenosine is produced. Adenosine helps muscles to adapt to exercise thus helping to prevent trauma. In addition, adenosine is also released in response to:

- Trauma of any kind
- Oxidative stress – where it helps to protect the brain

- Metabolic distress

Adenosine is found in all organs in the body where it has a diversity of functions including:

Kidneys – decreased blood flow and decreased production of rennin from the kidney

Lungs – constriction of airways

Liver – constriction of blood vessels and increased breakdown of glycogen to form glucose

Heart – decreased heart rate and has antiplatelet action and increased diameter of blood vessels in peripheral organs

Adenosine's numerous functions include:

- Relaxing vascular smooth muscle
- Regulating T cell proliferation and cytokine production - cytokines are small proteins that are secreted by cells of the immune system and have an effect on other cells.

- **In the form of adenosine monophosphate, relieving nerve pain including shingles**
- Inhibiting lipolysis

Now ATP is synthesised from fatty acids and protein from lean meats - chicken and turkey, for example - and also from fatty fish and nuts. However, as adenosine inhibits lipolysis, eating these foods – including chicken and turkey – have to potential to increase weight gain or the breakdown of fat for fuel.

This may take some time to get your head around. We are so used to hearing that turkey and chicken are ideal foods for weight loss and in some respects – within a calorie controlled diet - they may be. However, we cannot look at any food in the light of how many calories a portion contains. Any food has numerous nutritional substances contained within it and each of those will interact with an individual's genetic makeup and impact on many aspects of overall health.

As adenosine containing foods are essential for energy transfer then we should not seek to limit them from our diet. However, we need to be aware that too many may – in genetically susceptible people – carry the risk for unwanted weight gain which is difficult to lose. Reducing the amount of foods containing adenosine during calorie restriction – or blocking its action - would aid the breakdown of stored fat.

Adenosine monophosphate, in a study, has been found to be useful in treating the initial symptoms of shingles as well as post herpetic neuralgia. The study involved participants who were given 1000mg of AMP daily and those who were given placebos. At the end of the four-week trial of those who were given AMP, 88% were pain free compared to only 43% of those who were given placebos.

The actions of adenosine are antagonised by theophylline. The main source of theophylline is cocoa bean. Therefore, it is quite possible that eating foods containing theophylline may increase the pain of post herpetic neuralgia.

Agipenin (in parsley)

Agipenin is useful in alleviating neuropathic pain. Most people will eat parsley for its pain relieving effects. However, if you have the will you can crush the parsley and add it to a carrier oil and allow it to steep for two or three weeks in a darkened place before using it. Alternatively, you could crush some and add some DMSO to it for an hour or so before rubbing it into the affected part. It is messy but effective.

The whole parts of chamomile flowers can be used in a similar fashion.

With a little bit of thought a mixture of natural substances can be steeped in a carrier oil and used on the affected part. As each substance may have slightly differing actions on neuropathic pain then their combined effect should be far greater than using one substance alone. Meanwhile make sure that vitamin D intake is adequate and that vitamin C and zinc intake is increased.

Taurine as an NMDA Antagonist

We have already discovered that NMDA is a receptor for the neurotransmitter glutamate which once attached activates it.

Once it is activated it transmits pain.

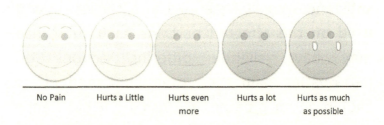

| No Pain | Hurts a Little | Hurts even more | Hurts a lot | Hurts as much as possible |

Once the NMDA receptor is activated by glutamate, it transmits pain

Taurine is an NMDA antagonist and can occupy the receptor thus preventing glutamate from doing so.

It is one of the few amino acids that is not used in protein synthesis and so is referred to as a 'nonessential' or 'conditionally' essential amino acid.

Taurine is an amino acid which is important in a number of metabolic processes going on in the body. For example, taurine has important functions in the brain and heart.

It is vital for nerve growth and has been considered beneficial for those with heart failure as it appears to reduce blood pressure.

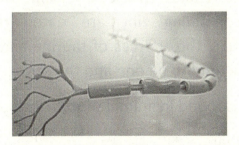

Taurine aids in the repair of damaged nerves

Its ability to repair damaged nerves is important in shingles. Damaged nerve fibres cannot carry signals from skin to brain efficiently. The signals may become exaggerated causing persistent and severe pain.

In some cases, the pain may be life-long. It is called post-herpetic neuralgia.

However, given taurine's ability to repair nerves and block the NMDA receptor, it is an excellent treatment for shingles.

Women have a greater requirement for taurine than men. The female hormone oestroedial blocks its synthesis in the liver.

Zinc is also vital to its use so it is important that foods containing zinc are eaten regularly. Fortunately, the sources of taurine and of zinc, generally tend to be one and the same.

Taurine is found in animal protein including:

- Meat
- Dairy
- Fish

It is especially rich in fish and the longevity of the Japanese is thought to be partly due to their diet which is rich in fish and therefore taurine.

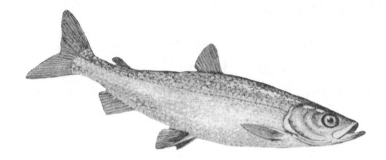

A diet high in fish would be particularly beneficial for those with shingles

Taurine can also be found in supplemental form online and in some health food shops.

It is generally in a fine granulated form and looks like castor sugar. A tiny measuring spoon is included with the amino acid. Be guided by the dose on the packet.

It doesn't have much of a taste so it can be stirred into a little water and drunk immediately.

This is probably the best way to take it if you have shingles since it is slightly more concentrated and more easily absorbed if taken on an empty stomach.

This is one of the benefits of having specific select amino acids to hand. They are absorbed, in the gut, almost immediately – within a couple of minutes – and when you are in pain that is important.

The effects of long term supplementation are not known with taurine but it is a useful supplement to take occasionally when pain, from any source, strikes.

A timely word is needed here though. When an easing of pain occurs which it will do with many of these supplements you must remember that pain is a symptom. Taking supplements to block the NMDA receptor will block the pain, sometimes dramatically, but the underlying reason for the disorder still needs to be addressed.

Shingles does not occur in the young primarily because immune systems have not become impaired as they do through age.

Knowing this imbues you with the knowledge that eating more healthily and using supplements wisely can help to boost a failing immune system.

It is in everyone's interest to learn about how the immune system works and to give it a little more attention than it usually gets.

Supplements are great in creating biological change which will help the body in dealing with symptoms.

So when we are looking at disease we must always bear in mind that

- The underlying causes must be addressed and
- Symptomatic relief given while the body is healing

Medication should never be started with the idea that it will be long term. It merely provides support and pain relief while you address the underlying causes of the condition through dietary changes.

The benefits of phenylalanine and tryptophan in treating pain

We have already learned that beneficial substances work by altering bodily processes. This is generally referred to as the pharmacological use of a substance.

When we look at drugs which address pain we find that there are two main types:

- Non-steroidal-anti-inflammatory drugs
- Steroid drugs
- Both of these have the potential for major negative side effects and in some cases can cause fatalities.

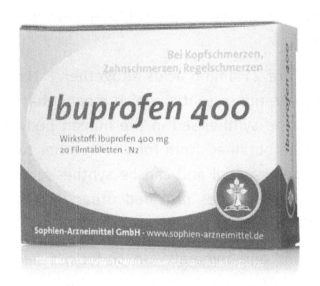

Ibuprofen is a non-steroidal anti-inflammatory drug

Amino acids like phenylalanine and tryptophan do not produce toxic side effects and have a lot to offer in terms of pain relief. They work in an entirely different way to ibuprofen which we shall look at shortly.

Firstly, it always helps to have a little understanding of the characteristics of all the amino acids. We simply could not live without them.

There are 21 amino acids altogether. Nine of these are non-essential which means that they cannot be synthesised in the human body and must be obtained from food. The other twelve are non-essential and can be synthesised from the essential ones provided other factors are available to aid this conversion.

Vitamins and minerals are co-factors and so, while we talk about non-essential amino acids as being less problematical to obtain, the reality is that they are very much reliant on the quality and quantity and variability of your diet.

You only have to be deficient in magnesium (and most people are) to find that one of the non- essential amino acids – which have unique properties – cannot be synthesised from its parent.

To take glycine, for example, it is the smallest of the non-essential amino acids but its importance in the body is breath taking.

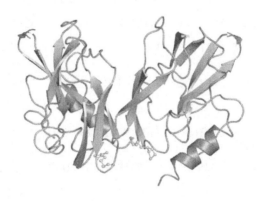

Glycine the small non-essential amino acid

Glycine forms nearly one quarter of connective tissue. That includes your skin, tendons and cartilage. Small and non-essential glycine may be but it is a very necessary amino acid.

Amino acids combine to produce enzymes and proteins necessary for growth and repair. They are needed to make hormones and keep your immune system going.

They regulate appetite and the sleep wake cycle and if you use them wisely they will address just about every ailment that you can get.

Phenylalanine is an essential amino acid which means that you must obtain it from food since your body cannot synthesise if from other substances.

It is the parent substance of tyrosine and dopamine, norepinephrine and adrenaline. All these are major players when it comes to good health.

Vitamins B6 and C are required for this biochemical conversion.

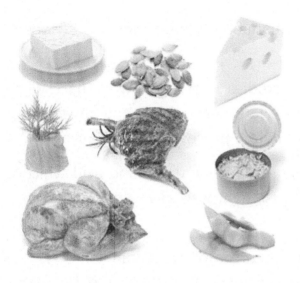

Phenylalanine is required by the thyroid for normal function but it is also required to maintain proper blood pressure and blood sugar levels, fat metabolism, heart rate and output and brain function.

It acts as an antidepressant, is useful in weight control and most importantly, for the subject matter of this book it is it enhances the body's own natural pain killers known as endorphins.

D phenylalanine is also capable of reducing inflammation and, in any cases of nerve damage, inflammatory processes will have been at work.

Certainly studies have shown that when endorphins were injected into the paws of rats the inflammatory processes were neutralised.

Tryptophan is an essential amino acid which is needed for the synthesis of vitamin B3 (nicotinic acid).

It is the precursor of serotonin which is the calming neurotransmitter but it also stimulates depressed individuals.

The less tryptophan people have the greater the degree of emotional disturbance.

A craving for carbohydrate generally occurs as a result of a deficiency of tryptophan.

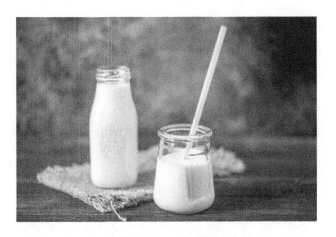

Milk is a good source of tryptophan

It also has powerful painkilling effects.

Phenylalanine and tryptophan are a formidable combination in pain control. Studies on 43 patients with intractable pain due to osteoarthritis were given 250mg of D-phenylalanine four times daily for five weeks.

Significant pain relief was noted.

Another study found that 7 out of 21 patients with chronic pain who took 750mg of D-phenylalanine over two weeks were able to stop all other pain killers due to a 50% reduction in pain levels. When you consider the potentially horrendous side effects of many painkillers then why D-phenylalanine is not used more often in analgesic medicine, I do not know.

Large doses – up to 2000mg (2g) –have been used before dental appointments.

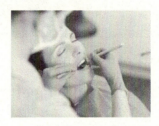

Phenylalanine is used as pain relief before dental appointments

It appears that those with chronic pain have low levels of natural endorphins. The ability of D-phenylalanine to retard the breakdown of endorphins ensures long pain relief for conditions.

This is especially important for conditions which involve nerve pain, like shingles, where there are few treatments available.

Tryptophan if taken with sugar in doses of 2-4g daily and no protein for 90 minutes also provides significant pain relieving effects.

Tryptophan is quite a large molecule and generally cannot enter the blood brain barrier as smaller molecules prevent it from doing so.

Therefore, tryptophan is much better taken at night before going to bed.

It is helpful if foods containing tryptophan and phenylalanine are increased in the diet when pain arises but clearly supplementation works quickly and provides the higher doses of amino acids that are needed at the time.

The recommended daily intake of phenylalanine is 30-40mg. Vegetarians and vegans are at risk of a deficiency as the main sources of phenylalanine are animal protein.

Two eggs will provide about one third of your daily requirement of this amino acid.

Many soda drinks contain phenylalanine if they are sweetened with aspartame. Aspartame is an artificial sweetener which is composed of two amino acids: aspartic acid and phenylalanine.

It also stands to reason that many artificial sweeteners are also a source of phenylalanine.

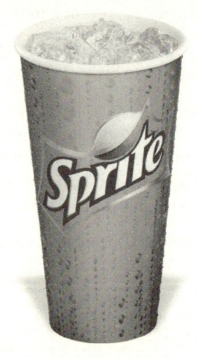

Soda is a source of phenylalanine

Tryptophan is also found mainly in animal sources of protein although peanuts are also a good source.

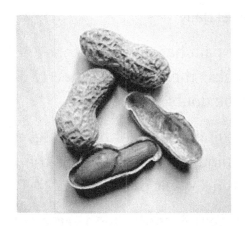

Peanuts are a good source of tryptophan

The recommended daily intake of tryptophan is approximately 500mg (half of one gram) and most people will obtain this in their diet.

Nevertheless, given the caution about its ability to cross the blood brain barrier when in the presence of other amino acids which are much smaller, it does beg the question of how much can actually be used by the body.

For pain relief D phenylalanine can be used thus:

750mg approximately 30 minutes before meals three times daily.

If relief of pain has not been considerable after three weeks, then for a further two days the dose can be doubled.

If this does not improve the pain levels, then D phenylalanine can be stopped as this is not the cause of the chronic pain.

Once the pain is controlled then phenylalanine can be stopped until there is a flare up of pain.

Please continue to look at the underlying causes of the pain and treat accordingly.

Quercetin

Quercetin is a plant flavonol from the flavonoid group of polyphenols. This means that it belongs to a large class of plant pigments which are full of micronutrients that are essential for health.

Quercetin is found in many fruits and vegetables with onions - and vegetables belonging to the onion family - being especially rich in it.

Quercetin is anti-inflammatory and antioxidant and is even able to reduce gouty arthritis related pain.

It is able to inhibit peripheral and spinal cord nociceptive mechanisms to reduce exercise induced muscle pain. It does this by stabilising the mast cell membrane which inhibits excessive histamine release.

More importantly, it is able to reduce neuropathic pain.

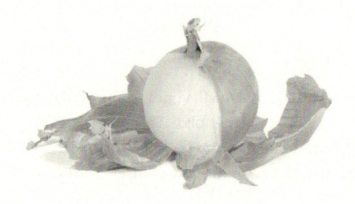

The humble onion is a great source of quercetin

The dorsal root ganglia consist of a group of cell bodies which emerge from between the vertebrae. They are responsible for the transmission of sensory messages to the central nervous system for a response.

Part of this transmission relies on a receptor called the $P2X_4$ receptor but quercetin inhibits this so that transmission of pain signals is reduced.

The reduction of pain is dose dependent. The maximum amount of quercetin that can be safely taken for pain varies and may take longer to control pain at lower doses.

However, doses of 1-30mg per kilogram of body weight have been taken for short periods with the lower doses taking up to 48 hours for an effect to be exerted

The larger doses have been found to work in 6-24 hours.

Other excellent sources of quercetin are:

- Garlic
- Apples
- Leeks

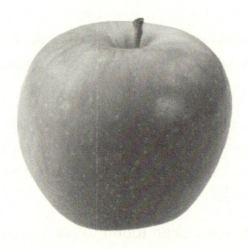

Although there are very few prescription-led treatments available for shingles, there is plenty we can do both in terms of avoiding it in the first place and secondly, addressing symptoms, through diet, should we be one of the unfortunate many who find it manifests itself in them.

Whenever disease strikes, it is a warning sign that we are suffering a deficiency of some sort so that our bodily systems are compromised in some way.

Shingles is not any different. It strikes when our immune system is impaired but this can always be addressed by a return to the principles of a good diet.

Thiamine (vitamin B1)

Thiamine is a much overlooked vitamin which has a wide range of applications. It is often ignored alongside its more well-known 'B' related cousins such as niacin and vitamin B12.

However, healing of nerves cannot take place without the presence of adequate amounts of thiamine and while many foods do contain thiamine it is easily destroyed during heating or in the water that food is cooked in.

There is a fat soluble form known as benfotiamine. It is easily converted to thiamine and is reputed to be more bio available thus increasing the amount of thiamine in the body.

A severe deficiency of thiamine is known as beriberi. The symptoms of beriberi are:

Swelling

Tingling

Burning sensation in limbs

Trouble breathing

Nystagmus (uncontrolled eyed movements)

Confusion and brain fog

Irritability

depression

abdominal discomfort

problems digesting carbohydrates

adrenal issues

inability to recall words.

Thiamine deficiency also provokes seizures.

The dry form of beriberi affects the central nervous system producing many of the symptoms described above. However, there is a wet form of beriberi where the predominant symptoms are:

High output congestive heart failure

Peripheral oedema

Tachycardia (rapid heartbeat)

Dilated cardiomyopathy

And, in practice if there is a deficiency of thiamine then there is likely to be an overlap of symptoms.

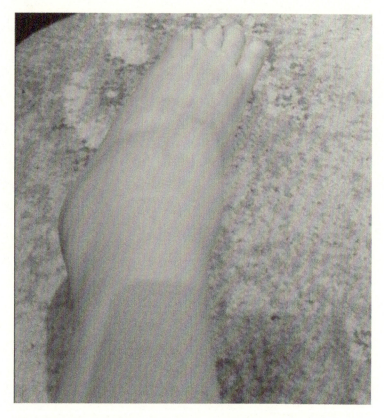

Peripheral oedema is a symptom of thiamine deficiency.

Thiamine is known as the 'ethical' vitamin due to its effect on the nervous system and mental behaviour. Indeed, individuals demonstrating aggressive behaviour, addictions or personality disorders are likely to be thiamine deficient.

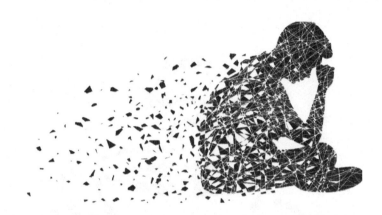

Brain fog is common with a thiamine deficiency

The above symptoms may be initiated or compounded by medications. One of the main culprits are diuretics with Furosemide (Lasix) appearing to be particularly mentioned in research papers.

Phenytoin (Dilantin), an anti-seizure medicine is also known to rapidly deplete thiamine in the body.

However, there are many foods and beverages that contain thiaminases – enzymes which destroy thiamine. The most notable ones are black tea and coffee but raw fish also contains a great deal of thiaminase that destroys this remarkable vitamin.

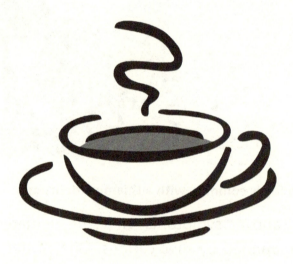

Coffee can deplete thiamine in the body

Stress also depletes thiamine rapidly and as I write this additional chapter to this book we are living through some very stressful events in the world.

On the plus side good sources of thiamine are to be found in a range of foods such as liver, whole wheat bread, other sources of whole grain, many vegetables and fortified foods. Nevertheless,

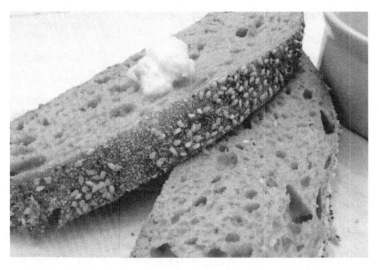

Whole wheat bread contains good amounts of thiamine

given that thiamine is easily destroyed it may be useful to supplement if tests suggest you are deficient, your diet is poor, you take certain medication you have a number of the afore mentioned symptoms or you have shingles or other nerve disorders.

Research shows that thiamine can be taken in high doses without any apparent negative side effects.

Having looked at the impact of a thiamine deficiency, how a deficiency may come about and what foods are high in this vitamin, our next step is to look at the positive impact that thiamine has on shingles.

B vitamins are generally taken in conjunction with other B vitamins. They work together well but thiamine in large doses can be used as an analgesic for neuropathic as well as non-neuropathic pain.

This dosage can be in the region of 1-4g with approximately 75% of patients receiving medications for their conditions gaining pain relief, shingles included.

Not every nutrient would be safe at doses stated to be many times higher than the Recommended Daily Intake (RDI) but thiamine appears to have no such disadvantage or be contraindicated at such high doses.

Thiamine is also required for myelin sheath maintenance. Studies have shown that when there is a thiamine deficiency then loss of myelin occurs but without any acute inflammation. Therefore, it can be understood that thiamine is needed for the synthesis, maintenance and repair of myelin which is damaged during shingles.

In addition, thiamine is required for the synthesis of a number of neurotransmitters such as serotonin and acetylcholine, the former well-known to reduce the strength of pain signals.

As thiamine is a vital cofactor in the conversion of carbohydrates   to cellular energy it also helps to provide energy to nerve cells.

The constant supply of energy is of vital importance because all nerve cells – including those in the brain - consume huge amounts of energy. It would be impossible to store the amount of energy that they need so thiamine must be available all the time.

Thiamine also has antioxidant properties and if there is sufficient available may prevent cell damage.

A small study [15]has also shown that the onset of shingles may be related to thiamine deficiency. Given thiamine's far reaching impact on   many systems in the body it is easy to see why.

Any nutrient is better taken in a well-rounded diet.   In the case of the B complex as they work

------

[15] https://pubmed.ncbi.nlm.nih.gov/24536615/

synergistically, then taking an individual B vitamin is not generally recommended. However, in the context of thiamine my recommendation, in the case of clear symptoms or signs of a deficiency is to supplement with thiamine while increasing foods which would contribute all the complex of B vitamins.

Whole wheat foods contain good amounts of most B vitamins. Many of them are fortified. Fortified niacin can be problematical for some though as it can cause indigestion, ulcers and gastritis – none of them pleasant at all to live with.

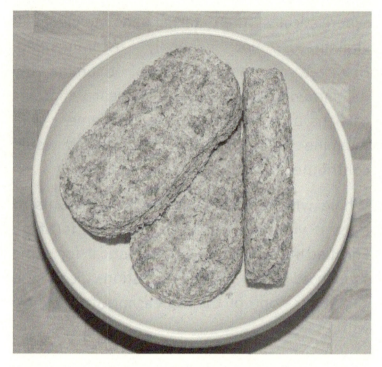

Whole wheat biscuits do contribute good amounts of the B complex. They are often fortified with iron and B vitamins.

By law a number of the B complex, iron and calcium in the form of calcium carbonate have been added for decades. This may pose problems for those who already have a healthy and substantial diet. These additives are added only to white flour. They are meant to replace the lost nutrients which you would find in the wholemeal varieties. I am not sure how that would work as during the making of any bread the heat used to bake bread will deplete some of the thiamine.

Liver is an excellent source of B complex provided it is lightly cooked and the water it is cooked in is used for gravy otherwise

You will lose much of the nutritional content of the food.

Liver is not eaten often nowadays which is a shame as it is superior in nutrients and could rightly be called a superfood.

When my children were little I would cook it and mince it to go into a Shepherd's pie. Lamb's liver has only a mild flavour and it was a favourite in our household.

The Recommended Daily Intake of thiamine is 100mg and it comes in that dosage generally.

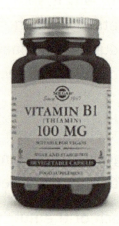

It is fairly inexpensive to buy considering the wide range of benefits it holds.

Now, looking at all the ways that can either help prevent, or treat shingles through repair or addressing neuropathic pain, it can be seen that a wide range of nutrients are involved in this process.

Shingles takes hold primarily because the immune system is compromised. It is likely to occur in the elderly because:

Their diets are not as rich and varied as they used to be. This could relate to the effort of cooking and the fact that many elderly living alone do not find satisfaction in cooking for one.

The ageing process makes it more likely that nutrients are not absorbed as efficiently as they were when an individual is younger.

Appetite diminishes so food, and nutrient, intake is reduced.

The amount of medications prescribed increases with age, not always wisely either. Some of these medications, like the Proton Pump Inhibitors, reduce the acidity of stomach acid so it is inefficient at breaking down food. This means that the nutrients can't be wholly extracted from them.

In order to address most of these issues, small but nutritionally dense meals that are very easy to prepare are recommended.

Medications may need to be reviewed. My husband, aged 77 years, is not on any medication and is a very happy and healthy individual. The fact that he does not take any prescribed medication is a source of amazement for his GP – whom he has never met – who periodically rings up to update their records.

As we go through life. Our dietary needs change. Sometimes we are slow to recognise this. We can eat bread without problem when we are young but as we age it begins to lie heavy on the stomach. We can eat what we like when we are young and not put an excess ounce of fat on but age changes all that.

Stress is also a contributing factor to shingles. Long term stress is known to deplete the immune system of the white immune system cells which seek out, attack and destroy infective agents such as that found in shingles.

I think, for the most part, that people have forgotten how to look after themselves or give themselves permission to rest or enjoy life.

Singles can be prevented and, if it does appear, its life can be curtailed rapidly and the chances of chronic neuropathic pain reduced.

We will now look at another of the vitamin B complex which has superior qualities when it comes to reducing nerve inflammation. This little known quality of riboflavin – vitamin B2- needs to be harvested more often.

Of course, we know that the incidence of shingles rises as we age. This should not come as a surprise to us due to the decreased capacity of absorption of nutrients which occurs in older age.

Riboflavin

Riboflavin is, as are all the other B vitamins, a water soluble vitamin. As such it is vulnerable to being destroyed during the preparation and cooking of food where it will leach out into the cooking water and normally be thrown away.

Riboflavin is found in a wide range of foods and is yet another of the B complex that is added to cereals and widely available as a dietary supplement at very reasonable cost.

Riboflavin is an essential component of two coenzymes:

a) Riboflavin -5-phosphate (Flavin mononucleotide)
b) Flavin adenine dinucleotide (FAD)

As with the b vitamins riboflavin is involved with energy production and the metabolism of fats, steroids and some medications.

When tryptophan is converted to niacin (vitamin B3) is requires the coenzyme FAD for this to be actioned.

The amino acid, homocysteine, a problematical amino acid which is only required briefly in the methionine cycle, cannot return to its normal place in this cycle without the presence of riboflavin.

Most riboflavin is absorbed in tiny amounts in the proximal small intestine and if not required only tiny amounts are stored in the heart and liver.

Some riboflavin is made in the large intestine but this very much depends on the gut flora which requires plant based material in order for riboflavin to be synthesised.

Meat does contain good amounts of riboflavin. For example, 3 ounces of beef contains approximately one third of the recommended daily intake of riboflavin. However, liver is by far superior as just one 3 ounce serving gives you twice the recommended dietary intake of riboflavin.

Riboflavin is rapidly deactivated by sunlight. The practise of using bottles to store milk was not helpful in this respect given that milk may be left on the doorstep for hours on end when the practise of having milk delivered by the milkman was common.

Now plastic containers are used and this offers some protection against ultra violet rays.

As only small amounts of riboflavin can be stored – and only for a short time - it is imperative that intake of riboflavin is at the forefront of your mind when addressing any inflammatory nerve disorders. You simply cannot be lackadaisical with your diet if this is the case.

Stress and some medications can play havoc with riboflavin levels. Diuretics are especially harmful given that they flush this nutrient out of the system rapidly. PPI's and other antacids do not create an environment where nutrients can be absorbed.

Other medications that may deplete riboflavin are:

Anticholinergic medications

Anticholinergic medications have a wide application and may be used to treat:

Motion sickness

Asthma

Spasms in the gastrointestinal tract

Some medications for depression including the tricyclic antidepressants – Nortriptyline, Amitriptyline, Imipramine and Desimpramine.

The phenothiazine type of antipsychotics reduces the amount of available riboflavin too. I have never yet known this impact on the bioavailability of riboflavin to be addressed when these medications are prescribed.

Methotrexate is commonly used to treat cancer and autoimmune diseases, especially, in the latter case, rheumatoid arthritis, However, methotrexate may make riboflavin less bioavailable than it would be without this prescription medicine.

A medication used for gout - Probenecid – reduces the amount of riboflavin that is absorbed in the gut.

Other problematical medications are Phenytoin (a seizure medication)

Doxorubicin – a medication for cancer which may deplete levels of riboflavin

.

While most medications interfere with the absorption of riboflavin, riboflavin can also interfere with the absorption of a broad spectrum antibiotic, tetracycline.

Riboflavin deficiency is not routinely tested for. As it is harder to maintain optimum levels as you age then it is worth considering whether to supplement if you have some more of the signs and symptoms of a riboflavin deficiency. Many of these appear unrelated but they are all manifestations of a riboflavin deficiency and include:

Sensitivity to light
Fatigue
Cracks and sores around the mouth (angular stomatitis)
Eye fatigue
Sore throat
Swollen throat
Magenta-coloured and swollen tongue
Thyroid hormone insufficiency
Cheilosis - swollen cracked lips
Itchy and red eyes
Hair loss
Reproductive problems
Degeneration of the liver
Degeneration of the nervous system

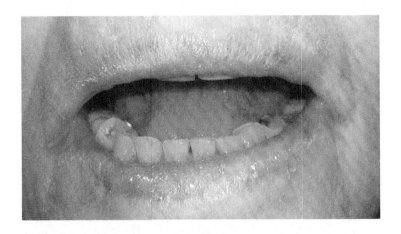

Angular stomatitis found in riboflavin deficiency, notice the cracks at the side of the mouth

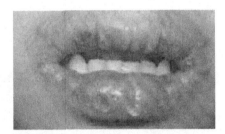

Cheilosis – lips are swollen dry and cracked, flaky or scabbing over

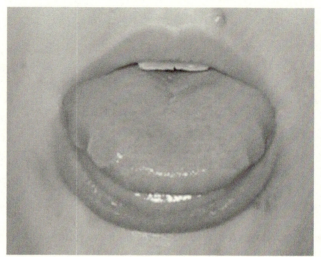

Swollen tongue

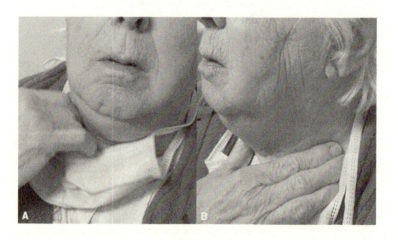

Swollen throat in riboflavin deficiency

As the symptoms of riboflavin deficiency are so overt, then it is worth memorising them. Riboflavin deficiency can be fleeting so that relapses and remittance can occur with regularity – none of which is good for health. Subclinical nutrition of riboflavin occurs frequently, damaging health but maybe not showing signs as can be seen above.

As with any nutritional deficiency, the range of symptoms any individual may have - or the signs that they may show - may differ widely due to genetic variation. Therefore, out of a range of say, ten symptoms and signs, one individual may show symptoms 1, 5 and 7 and another may show signs and symptoms, 2, 3, 5, 8, 9, 10.

It has also to be born in mind that specific nutrients are not activated in isolation from other nutrients. A case in point is   that thiamine needs magnesium in order for it to be used. Therefore, if you have identified a riboflavin deficiency and are resolved to supplement with riboflavin, then it may be useful to also take a good all round supplement which supplies all the trace minerals and vitamins to support the specific supplement for the known deficiency.

I hope that I have now shown that Shingles manifests itself as a sign of an unhappy immune system but that this can be identified and corrected hopefully before symptoms manifest themselves.

Even if full blown shingles develops then early treatment can shorten or prevent the pain associated with this condition.

I am committed to supporting small businesses whose ethos closely follows that of mine where caring for health through natural means is of paramount importance.

I am happy to recommend SkinKiss, a small business whose ethos is as follows:

It's all about living a natural life.

Natural bath and body products with NO parabens, SLS, Mineral Oil, Palm Oil or synthetic fragrances.

Cruelty-free & vegan too and packaged in recycled cardboard.

Here at SkinKiss we believe that what we put ON our bodies is as important as what we put IN our bodies.

We love all things natural and only source & use the best ingredients, including organic where possible.

Nature provided us with so many amazing plants & we love to turn them into bath and body gorgeousness.

There are 20 different fragrances in soaps including lavender and lemongrass, shampoo bars, bath soaks and so much more all designed to help you reduce the stress in your life.

Skinkiss can be found on Twitter, Facebook and has an online store which can be found here.

https://skinkiss.org.uk/

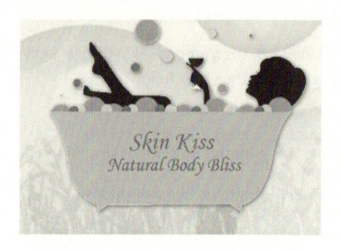

That's my present list sorted, then.

Other books on a wide range of health related subjects by this author can be found here:

https://authorcentral.amazon.co.uk

https://www.amazon.com/~/e/B07BPQZ5CD

and include:

Other books by this author include:

- The EDS and Hypermobility Syndrome Diet
- Alleviating Symptoms of EDS
- Gastroparesis
- The EDS recipe book
- The Lipoedema Diet
- The Lymphoedema Diet: reverse and repair lymphatic damage
- The Anti Virus Diet
- The Asthma Diet
- The Reluctant Bowel
- The MND Diet
- Why we live longer with higher cholesterol levels
- A dietary connection for MACS, POTS and EDS
- Identity: a self-exploration workbook *
- Journey Through Pneumonia
- https://www.amazon.co.uk/dp/B07TB HMV6N

*This book can be used alone or in small group work and is an excellent resource for those who are 'people helpers.'

Among many others

They are available on Amazon

Lynne has written a semi-autobiographical trilogy.

While this trilogy is available on kindle and paperback on Amazon, it may be cheaper to buy from the link below.

They may be obtained off the publisher's website, in paperback form, where they are more reasonably priced.

https://www.shieldcrest.co.uk/?s=lynne+d+m+noble++

.

A percentage of royalties from the sale of this book is allocated for charitable purposes   like The Exodus Project below. Thank you for your support.

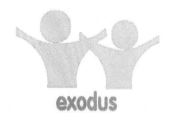

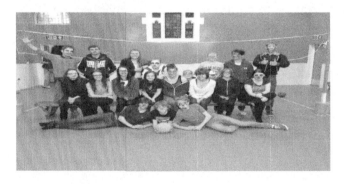

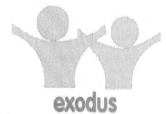

Exodus has been impacting the lives of children and young people in less advantaged communities for 20 years. Through a unique model of working, we build trusting relationships that create firm foundations for growing aspirations and regenerating communities. We target the most disadvantaged communities, trying to get kids to make the right choices for their lives.

We have learned that none of this will be achieved without long term commitment to the children and their families in these communities. Superficial remedies to deep rooted problems will only have short term impact. We are regarded as friends and not workers in the areas where we work. Our work is long established and our reputation for consistency and commitment is unquestioned. So what do we do?

We run mid-week activity clubs in the heart of the less advantaged communities of Barnsley. We bus in equipment and volunteers, to join local people in delivering exciting and fast moving activity programmes for the local kids. The programmes are great fun, as well as educational. We do dance, drama, craft, music, sports and games to entertain and energise. We also talk to the kids about the issues going on in their communities. So, if the local allotments have been broken into, or kids have been playing football on the bowling green again, we can discuss anti-social behaviour and attitudes with examples that the local young people identify with.

As well as activity clubs and home visits we take the kids away on activity weekends. We have our own activity centre, known as Jenny's Field, which we use for these weekend retreats. Jenny's Field is a home from home and a place of refuge and encouragement for so many children and young people.

The final aspect of our work might generally be termed "community partnerships". We don't want to work in isolation and we partner with parents and carers, local residents' associations, the police, housing authorities, schools and others to ensure a coordinated approach to issues on the estates.

Perhaps the most rewarding aspect of our work is the development of junior volunteers. Many of the young people who come through the activity clubs structure continue their involvement with us as leaders in the clubs where they were once members. Over the years we have nurtured hundreds of young people, sustaining relationships with them throughout their turbulent teenage years. Joe says it best:

"I very quickly fell into the family of Exodus. At such a young age nothing in my life was certain, but I knew that I belonged here. I've gone from a gobby little kid, who used to spend hours in a porch, to a not much bigger adult with a remarkable story to tell, of how God has guided and supported me and lead me down the right path, when it would have been so easy to stray."

Facebook: TheExodusProjectBarnsley

www. exodusproject.org.uk

Made in the USA
Las Vegas, NV
13 January 2024

84310328R00080